Essential Strategies For Academic Success

By Ben Kim, D.C.

Library and Archives Canada Cataloguing in Publication Data

Kim, Ben 1973 –
8 essential strategies for academic success / Ben Kim.
ISBN 0-9737939-1-0

1. Academic achievement. 2. College students--Health and hygiene. I. Title. II. Title: Eight essential strategies for academic success.

LB2395.K36 2005 378.1'98 C2005-905104-3

Dr. Ben Kim Natural Health Solutions, Inc.
P.O. Box 20185
Barrie, Ontario L4M 6E9
Canada
http://drbenkim.com

Printed in Canada

Contents

Also written by Ben Kim:

Experience Your Best Health: A complete guide to taking care of your health from the inside out

Introduction

My Academic Journey

Like many kids of my generation, I was raised to believe that my main mission in life was to get the highest grades possible in school. My dad raised me to be supremely confident in my abilities. Even before I set foot into my first kindergarten class, he had me convinced that I was the smartest kid in the world; maybe not the healthiest way to prepare a child to be humble and work well with others, but this is the mindset that likely developed for my father as a result of his poverty-stricken childhood in post-war Korea.

Early on, my dad's lessons and mindset produced good results. I studied pretty hard throughout elementary, junior high, and high school, and never found it too difficult to get good grades. As I got ready to go to university, I was feeling pretty good about my chances of getting into medical school and becoming the doctor that my parents hoped I would become.

Little did I know how unprepared I was for the competition that awaited me in university. Looking back, I can say that I was pretty innocent, thinking that I'd meet good friends, play some sports, study hard, get good grades, and become a doctor. I really had no idea how well prepared many of my classmates were to get top-notch grades and make it to medical school. It was a world of private school and top public school students from all over Canada and Hong Kong whose entire high school careers, it seemed, had been geared towards getting the grades needed to get into medical school.

I should share a little background on the school system in Canada for those of you who aren't familiar with it. Here in Canada, the government provides a lot of financial support to its universities and colleges, far more than any private universities receive from the federal government in the States.

Because of the large government subsidies involved, universities in Canada are less business oriented than private schools in the States. While tuition at some private universities in the States can cost upwards of $20,000.00 USD in tuition per year, almost all Canadian universities cost around $5,000.00 CAD in tuition per year. All of this means that there are fewer positions available in Canadian universities, since it's not the case that anyone with average grades and enough money can enter the program of his or her choice. This, of course, translates to more intense competition to get into medical, dental, and law schools in Canada than to get into the same schools in the States.

Getting back to my introduction to academics in university, I was in mild shock to receive B's and even a C on my mid-terms. Although slightly discouraged, I was confident that all I needed to do was work even harder for the rest of the semester to get the higher grades that I was used to.

As you can probably guess, things didn't get better. My grades continued to be average as the year wore on, regardless of how hard I studied. By the end of the school year, I had to face reality; if things continued to go the way they were going, I would have to go the long route – B.Sc., M.Sc., and PhD. – to have a chance of getting into medical school in Canada. And God knew that my parents couldn't afford to send me to medical school in the States, which was a viable option for other students in Canada whose parents could afford to pay the big bucks that U.S. schools charge.

For the rest of my time at the University of Toronto, I continued to do my best, taping and repeatedly listening to lectures, writing endless notes, and staying up until 2 in the morning on a regular basis, poring over my textbooks. But my grades remained the same.

As I approached the beginning of my third year of university, I had a decision to make. Was I going to stick around and turn into a professional student, pay tuition, build debt, and not make income for the next ten to fifteen years? Or was I going to be bold and move in a different direction? A trip to the local career center helped make up my mind. In reading through alternative careers for health science majors, a pamphlet on chiropractic caught my attention. The description that I read on chiropractors – primary health care providers who use only natural methods – was very appealing, especially since I had all of the pre-requisites needed to begin right away.

Within a few months, I found myself in the suburbs of Chicago, where I began a four-year program that would lead to a Doctor of Chiropractic degree. Grateful for the fresh start, I was determined to learn from my hard times at the University of Toronto and become the most effective and clear-minded student that I could be. I thought carefully about what I could change about my study habits to improve my ability to understand new subjects and my performance on exams. Even before my first class, I spent more than one whole week doing nothing but devising a plan on how to do this.

With my carefully constructed plan and focus, I ended up carrying a 4.0 GPA for much of the four-year program, despite working 20 hours a week as a research fellow for much of it. I deliberately let my GPA slide to 3.86 in the final three academic semesters because I was too shy to take on the responsibility of giving the valedictory address.

I'm not sharing this story to be boastful. I'm sharing this story because I came to realize that anyone can become a super effective learner and high achiever in school if they adopt a few key strategies and follow a well-designed study plan.

If there's one lesson that stands out above the rest from my years as a formal student, it is this: how much you study is not nearly as important as how you study. You can learn and remember new subjects more effectively in 30 minutes than you can in weeks if you have the right approach.

That's what this book is about; how to avoid all the mistakes I made early on in my academic career and how to study in a way that will allow you to learn new topics with a level of understanding that will make it natural for you to remember these topics for many years.

I originally intended to save the material in this book for my own children when they reached an appropriate age. But I changed my mind because it occurred to me one day that there are probably only a few people out there who are earnestly looking for this information *and* are willing to apply it to their studies. I want this book to be available to these people. I hope that you are one of them.

Strategy Number One:

Learn It to Teach It

Strategy number one, learn it to teach it, is the single most important key to becoming an exceptional learner and experiencing academic success. Whenever you sit down to learn or review a subject, take on the mindset that you have to teach it to someone younger than you the next day. This will allow you to learn more in 30 minutes of studying than you can in hours or weeks without this mindset.

When you take on the mindset of having to teach a new subject to someone the next day, your mind will be focused on truly understanding the subject. This is the only way to learn a subject in a way that will allow you to remember it for years. If you can't explain a subject to others in a way that is easy for them to understand it, then you either don't fully understand the topic, or you need to work at clarifying your explanation. When you go through this process, you will own the subject in question.

This is why it is especially helpful to take on the mindset that you have to teach each new subject that you learn *to someone who is younger than you,* preferably a child. Clearly, you have to understand a subject really well to be able to explain it well enough for a child to understand it.

The mindset of thinking like a teacher means that you should practice teaching new material out loud. You should pretend that a student is listening when you teach the material that you just learned. If you prefer to study in a library or somewhere else that doesn't allow for you to speak out loud, you should at least talk through your explanations inside your head. Another option is to write it out in your own words, although this can take a lot more time than just talking out loud or talking it through in your head.

It's fine to use paper, pencil and pen to jot down notes, work through problems, and do anything else that will help you understand the subject at hand. What you must be careful *not* to do is turn note-making into a project in itself. Many students are more interested in having a neat looking binder and beautiful notes and diagrams than actually understanding the material. I should know – I used to be one of them.

If you write notes with the primary purpose of creating a beautiful notebook or binder, that's probably all you'll have left at the end of the semester. If you write notes to help you understand the material well enough to teach it to someone else, you'll keep that information in your noggin for many years if not the rest of your life. Put another way; don't worry so much about how much time you have logged at your desk or how many pages of notes you have written. The bottom line is how much you have truly understood of the topic you are studying, regardless of how much time you spent studying it.

Here's an added bonus to studying with the mindset of trying to understand the material well enough to teach it: doing so will help you remember the information come exam time, *even if you never end up understanding it.* That's right, if you rack your brain hard enough trying to understand a difficult concept or one that is poorly explained by your teacher or textbook, your efforts to figure it out will cause you to remember the topic well enough to answer any test question about it. When you run into this scenario while taking an exam, you may find yourself thinking, "Well, this still doesn't make any sense, but I know exactly what they're looking for."

Strategy Number One:

Learn It to Teach It

Strategy Number Two:

Be Comfortable While You Study

Mix up your studying locations. You don't have to sit at your desk every time that you study. For some people, studying in the same location every single time can be helpful in establishing a routine and mindset for learning. For others, effective studying requires first and foremost that they are as physically comfortable as possible. There's nothing wrong with spending 15 minutes reading and writing at your desk and then another 15 minutes reading while lying on your side in bed. Some of my most effective study sessions occurred first thing in the morning while I was still lying in bed.

Another strategy I used to make my study sessions comfortable was to sit or lie down to read a new concept, and then teach it out loud while I slowly walked around my room. I was amazed by how effectively I could think and teach out loud when I slowly paced back and forth.

If you find yourself drifting to other thoughts or reading the same paragraph more than two or three times because you weren't paying attention, get up and do something else for 5-15 minutes. Go lie down and stretch out your body. Close your eyes for a few minutes and let you mind and body relax. When you feel mentally and physically refreshed, get back to your books and try it again.

Strategy Number Two:

Be Comfortable While You Study

Strategy Number Three:

Take Advantage of the Best Time to Study

Don't miss the best time to absorb new information: right after you wake up. After a period of quality sleep, whether it's a whole night's rest or a solid nap, your brain will have more blood available to absorb ideas and concepts that it won't be as easily able to grasp when your body is tired or busy spending its blood and energy on digesting a big meal.

The worst time to study is after a big meal. Did you know that a large portion – some physiologists say as much as 50 percent - of your blood supply must go to your digestive organs after each meal? With so much blood going to your digestive tract, there's little left over in your circulation for optimal brain function. There's no question that you are far better off resting for 30 to 90 minutes after a big meal than you are hitting the books again right after a meal.

If you find yourself going over a new topic repeatedly without developing the feeling that you truly understand it, save it for the next time you wake up from a solid nap or full night's rest. I owe much of my success in chiropractic school to this one simple technique.

Strategy Number Three:

Take Advantage of the Best Time to Study

Strategy Number Four:

Make Each Class Count

One of the best habits that you can develop as a student is to go to class and pay attention. It amazes me how many students make the effort to show up to class, only to sit there daydreaming or fooling around. I remember one fellow who always sat beside me in as many classes as possible so that he could copy down my notes while I wrote down what I felt was important from the professor's lectures. He could pay attention enough to copy my notes, but he just couldn't pay attention enough to listen to the professor himself.

Paying attention in class is the very best way to really learn what's important to the teacher. All teachers have areas of their required textbooks and teaching material that they like to emphasize over other areas. You won't learn which areas these are without paying attention in class. Plus, if you truly pay attention in class and understand the material as it is being presented, it will make things much easier when you go to review the material later on and prepare for an exam.

Also, if you pay attention in class, whenever your teacher runs across a point that you don't understand, you can address your confusion in the moment. Don't be afraid to ask about anything that you aren't sure about. So many students are so afraid of looking dumb that they end up sitting there, lost in a daze. Once you miss one important point in a lecture, you could be lost for the rest of the lecture, or quite possibly, for the rest of the semester. If you want to do as well as possible in school, you **must** stay on top of each point of every class. So what if some students snicker about you being a teacher's pet or a nerd. Asking questions in class about points that you don't understand is absolutely essential to saving time and getting good grades. By asking questions in class, you can clear up a point that you don't understand within 20 seconds rather than frustrate yourself for hours trying to understand it in the wee hours of the morning the night before an exam.

Not only should you ask questions without hesitation, you should be sure to sit at or near the front of the classroom. When I was formal student, I sat all over the place. I can tell you with certainty that it was easiest for me to concentrate and understand new lessons whenever I sat at the front of the class.

One last point about getting the most out of your classes: in almost all cases, it is best not to tape your lectures. It takes a lot of time to re-listen to lectures on tape. You can effectively review material from a one-hour lecture in about 15 minutes by going through your notes. Listening to a tape will take you close to the full hour, depending on how much you fast forward through it. Also, I have noticed that people who tape lectures tend to lose focus more easily than those who don't tape lectures in class, probably because they feel that if they miss something, they have their tape to listen to later on. Make things easy on yourself – stay focused in class and save countless hours outside of class.

One way to help you stay focused in class is to make it a habit to preview new material before it is presented in class. I'm not talking about poring over the new material and becoming an expert. Just a quick read-through is often enough to give you a solid idea of what your teacher will be talking about that day. Often times, it is easy to sit through a one-hour lecture and not remember a single point because you just weren't clear on the big picture of what your teacher was trying to teach that day. Knowing the overall theme of each lesson before sitting your bum down in a classroom chair can make a huge difference in your ability to learn things the right way from the beginning.

Most classes begin each semester with the teacher handing out a syllabus that outlines what each lecture will be about. If you find that your teacher doesn't follow the syllabus very closely, be sure to talk with him or her at the end of each class or week to find out which sections of your textbook or class notebook are going to be covered during the next few days. Previewing class lessons in this way is another strategy that sounds like a ton of work, but adopting this strategy will save you more hours than you can imagine. It will also improve your performance on exams, which will give you more confidence, which in turn will strengthen your resolve to continue with this strategy – a nice little cycle to create.

Another way to squeeze the most out of each class: review the material that you covered in class later that day or night. If you tried hard to understand the material in class, reviewing it during a spare period or at night will take you very little time. A nightly review is an excellent time to work through any points that are still not completely clear to you. Be sure to jot these points down in a place where you won't lose it, so that you can ask the teacher about it as soon as possible. Doing a nightly review for each of your classes sounds like it will require a lot of time and energy. The truth is that doing so will save you incredible amounts of time and energy. If done properly, it shouldn't take more than an average of around 15 minutes to review the lessons of each one hour class. The more you paid attention in class that day, the quicker your review will be.

Strategy Number Four:

Make Each Class Count

Strategy Number Five:

Learn How to Write Exams Effectively

While you're writing an exam, after reading through a question, if you aren't confident about how to figure out the answer immediately, move on to the next question. Proceed in this way until you answer all of the questions on the exam that are relatively easy for you. Only then should you go back to the harder questions and take your time in trying to figure them out. If you try to tackle the hard questions first or just stick to the order in which the exam is presented, you could lose valuable time and make mistakes on or not even get to easier questions.

If you are taking a test that involves multiple choice options, as you read through each option, be sure to cross out choices that you are absolutely sure are wrong. Sounds like an obvious step to take, but many students don't do this and waste valuable time re-reading answers that they know are irrelevant. Also, if you start to run short on time, you will increase your chances of guessing the correct response if you have clearly eliminated incorrect choices beforehand.

Speaking of exam-writing techniques, let's not ignore the obvious when it comes to math and science courses in high school and especially in college and university. Old exams can be like gold. You may already know how this works. Many teachers and professors use the same or similar questions semester after semester, year after year. Generous classmates share old tests that they've received from upper classmen. Stingy classmates go to great lengths to hide old tests that they've collected and swear up and down that they don't have anything.

If getting the highest grades that you possibly can is important to you, then you owe it to yourself to ask around and be sure that you have access to the same old tests that everyone else does. You may not need to look at them to do well, but why put yourself at a disadvantage? Not looking at old tests while everyone else does is like starting 20 meters behind the start line in a 100 meter sprint. I do not consider using old tests as cheating. Going over old tests can help you figure out which parts of the study material you understand well, and which parts you still aren't clear on.

Getting a hold of old tests is one thing. Knowing how to use them to study effectively is an entirely different matter.

When I first started looking at old tests, I saved them for after I spent hours upon hours studying my textbooks and notes first. After a while, it became obvious to me that a much better approach was to read through the old tests first. Doing so gave me an excellent idea of how I needed to study my textbooks and notes. Looking at the tests first helped me figure out which areas I really needed to focus on, and the perspective from which the professor or teacher thought about the material at hand.

If you take my advice on this, be sure *not* to fall into a huge trap that the majority of students do in spending the bulk of your study time on these old tests and just memorizing the answers. If the old tests are in multiple choice format, as you read through each option, you should be able to figure out why the correct answer is in fact, correct, and why the remaining options are incorrect. If you can't figure out exactly why an answer is correct or incorrect, you need to study your notes or talk with your professor until you do.

Strategy Number Five:

Learn How to Write Exams Effectively

Strategy Number Six:

Be Respectful and Real With Your Teachers

Get to know your teachers and professors. They are people, just like you and your parents. Realize that they probably have all the same financial stressors, relationship challenges, and personal insecurities that most people do.

You probably know full well how hard it is to decide what you want to do for the rest of your life. Your teachers most likely went through the same struggles, and while some of them may be happy with their teaching careers, some of them may not be. Learning to see your teachers as real people with the same problems, hopes, and dreams that the rest of us have can help you stay fresh and focused when you run into a class or teacher that you just don't connect with.

Whenever you interact with your teachers, be sincere and real. You don't need to butter them up with compliments or fear them as though they own the land you live on. Be genuine and treat them with respect, and you will likely have a student-teacher relationship that will help you be an effective student.

Strategy Number Six:

Be Respectful and Real With Your Teachers

Strategy Number Seven:

Learn How to Write Effectively

Math, science, and subjects that require a lot of memorization like history always came easier to me than subjects that required a lot of writing. My sisters, both teachers with multiple post secondary degrees in English, will tell you that I'm far from being a natural born talent when it comes to writing. Sure, there are some days when the words seem to flow easily, but there are also days when writing a single paragraph can be a long and frustrating process.

Despite my lack of natural writing ability, there are a few tips that I have learned over the years that have made it possible for me to complete several written projects, including this book. I hope that the following tips on effective writing are as helpful to you as they are for me.

1. **Get clear first, brainstorm second.** Before you write anything, get clear on the topic and what your piece will be about. Once you are

clear on the topic, spend some time jotting down any and all thoughts that come to your mind about that topic. Brainstorm. Let your creative powers flow and don't hesitate to write down every idea that enters your head, no matter how silly or dumb it seems in the moment. A good brainstorming session can last anywhere from a few minutes to a few hours. Once you feel like you are done with this process, take a look at what you have written down. Keep the ideas that you feel are relevant to the topic you are writing on. Cross out the rest.

2. **Make an outline.** Use your list of ideas to create an outline. All you need are a few words or a short sentence or two to describe each major section of the piece that you will be writing.

3. **Write a first draft ...quickly!** Use your outline to begin writing each section. The key to writing your first draft is to let the words flow naturally. Don't worry about making each sentence perfect. Write as you would talk. Be natural. Don't use words that you wouldn't use in real life.

4. **Take a break, then go back and edit.** Once you get through a natural, free flowing draft of your piece, take a break. Don't try to fill in the details and edit your first draft right away. Take a few hours off, or take the whole day off. Once you have given yourself a break from your work, you can go back and fill in the details and make the changes that you want. Taking some time off before this editing process will make it easier for you to notice areas that need polishing than it will be if you try to edit your first draft right after you write it.

5. **Take another break and edit one last time.**

   Once you get through with the editing process, give yourself another break from your work – an hour or even a day. Then, read through it one more time, this time looking to see how well your material flows from section to section, and if you have successfully stayed on track without going off on unnecessary tangents.

Strategy Number Seven:

Learn How to Write Effectively

Strategy Number Eight:

Use Optimal Nutrition to Boost Your Brain Power

Have you ever noticed that there are times when you can absorb new ideas and solve problems with absolute ease, and how there are other times when no matter how hard you try, you can't stay focused or solve the simplest of problems?

Other than how well rested you are, the most important factor that can influence your brain power and ability to focus and solve problems is what you choose to eat on a regular basis. If you consistently make poor food choices, you can expect to have poor focus, poor memory, and low capacity to understand new subjects. If you consistently make good food choices, you will boost your brain's capacity to absorb new information, solve problems, and perform to the best of your ability on exams.

Most people want to believe that there is a list of three or five specific foods that they can eat on a regular basis that will boost their brain power and grades. Anyone who offers such a list would be doing you a disservice.

There are no short cuts to providing optimal nutrition to your brain and body, just like there are no short cuts to anything that is worthwhile in life. The only way to use nutrition to your advantage as a student is to make healthy food choices on a regular basis. In other words, there is no magical supplement that will counteract the negative effects of wolfing down candy bars and soda. There are no miracle foods that can erase the burden that a regular diet of junk and processed foods will put on your brain and body.

Before we look at what your overall diet should look like, let's address a few important fundamentals:

1. **Chew your foods until liquid.** Doing so will take a tremendous amount of burden off of your digestive organs. Your teeth and jaws are designed to *mechanically* break down the

foods you eat into smaller particles. Your digestive organs – your stomach, small intestine, liver, gall bladder, and pancreas – are designed to *chemically* break down these smaller food particles into even smaller nutrients (amino acids, triglycerides, and glucose) that are able to enter your blood stream and be used by your body for energy and construction of new cells. If you don't chew your foods until liquid, you will put unnecessary burden on your digestive organs to break down large food particles into small nutrients, work that your digestive organs are not designed to do on a regular basis. If you put this unnecessary strain on your digestive organs on a regular basis, your body will have to spend an excessive amount of your blood supply and energy on digestion. This, of course, leads to less available blood supply and energy for your brain and thinking capacity.

2. **After you eat a good-sized meal, give your mind and body a half hour to an hour of rest.** Doing so will allow your body to devote the bulk of its blood supply to efficiently and completely digest your meal. Running around doing errands or trying to cram more information into your brain right after a big meal is likely to result in poor digestion, which will lead to your body having to spend more energy dealing with incompletely digested food in the hours that follow. This is a sure way of promoting poor focus and decreased learning capacity.
3. **Strive to eat fresh, natural foods most of the time.** What's the definition of fresh and natural? Just look to eat foods that you would find in a garden, orchard, on a farm, or in the wild. Eating fresh and natural foods on

regular basis is the best way of promoting optimal digestion, which will in turn leave your body with as much energy as possible to feed your brain and learning capacity.

With these three fundamentals in mind, the following is a list of healthy foods that can promote optimal brain function and health:

Fruits

- Berries – blueberries, raspberries, and strawberries
- Cherries
- Fresh figs or dried figs that have been soaked for a few hours
- Avocado
- Coconut
- Mango
- Papaya
- Apples
- Pears
- Watermelon and other melons

It is best not to eat too many fruits, as the natural sugars in fruits can cause you to feel sleepy in the long run, just like table sugar and other sweeteners can. Two to five servings of fruit per day is just fine for most people. Fruit juices should be avoided most of the time, as they can put the same stress on your body that sugar water can. Dried fruit should not be eaten regularly. When you do eat dried fruits, be sure to soak them in water for a few hours before eating to dilute their concentrated sugars.

Vegetables

- Romaine, red leaf, and green leaf lettuce
- Celery
- Carrots
- Tomatoes
- Zucchini
- Spinach
- Swiss chard
- Kale
- Cabbage
- Green beans
- Peas

Vegetables should make up at least 50 percent of your diet. They provide an abundance of nutrients and are easy to digest for most people. If you have trouble eating a lot of raw vegetables, try them steamed or cooked with extra virgin olive oil or coconut oil over a low to medium temperature. One key to eating lots of vegetables on a regular basis is to make tasty and healthy dressings to go along with them. See the recipe section at the back of this book for a variety of delicious and healthy dressings.

Whole Grains

- Brown rice
- Quinoa
- Buckwheat
- Millet
- Oatmeal

Strive to soak your whole grains overnight in water and drain them before cooking the next day. This will help to prevent mineral deficiencies that can occur if you eat whole grains that are not soaked before being prepared to eat.

If you are going to eat bread a few times a week, be sure to use a dense, whole grain bread that isn't so soft that you can squish a whole loaf down to the size of a tennis ball. With bread, the grittier, the better. When making a sandwich with a gritty, whole grain bread, add lots of baby field greens or baby spinach to help ensure that vegetables remain the main staple of your diet.

Nuts and Seeds

- Raw walnuts
- Raw almonds
- Raw pecans
- Raw, organic peanuts
- Raw sunflower seeds

Like whole grains, raw nuts and seeds should be soaked in water overnight and drained and dried in the morning before being eaten. If you forget to soak your nuts from time to time, it's fine to go with unsoaked nuts, as they are far better for your health than candy bars and other processed foods.

It is best to eat no more than about two handfuls of raw nuts and seeds per day, one handful if you experience bloating or gas with two handfuls. Don't forget to chew nuts and seeds until liquid.

Legumes

- Chickpeas (hummus)
- Black beans (black bean dip)
- Kidney beans
- Small red beans
- Pinto beans
- Navy beans
- Lima beans
- Miso soup and paste (fermented soy beans)

Ideally, it is best to buy dry legumes, soak them in water overnight, and then to cook them for an hour or two before eating. Because a student's life does not always permit enough free time to go through this simple but time-consuming process, canned legumes are acceptable. Be sure to drain canned legumes of their preservative-laden liquid and then to give them a thorough rinse to remove as much of the liquid as possible. If time permits, you can dunk them in boiling water for a minute and drain again to ensure that little or no preservatives remain in contact with the legumes.

If you make a batch of hummus out of chickpeas (see the recipe section at the back of this book), once a week and keep it in an airtight container in the refrigerator, you'll have a healthy and delicious protein-dense paste to eat with salads, steamed vegetables, and whole grain sandwiches.

Clean Animal Foods

- Organic eggs from free range birds
- Organic yogurt, but only if you don't experience bloating, gas, diarrhea, earaches, nasal congestion, and skin eruptions within hours of eating it
- Organic butter
- Wild salmon
- Anchovies
- Sardines
- Free-range, organic chicken
- Grass-fed beef
- Grass-fed lamb
- Any kind of wild game

Whenever you eat clean animal foods, you should limit your serving size to about the size of a deck of cards or less, and eat it with lots of vegetables. The antioxidants and fiber in vegetables will help to prevent free radical damage and constipation, respectively, which can result from eating too many animal foods in one sitting or on a regular basis. In general, my opinion is that most people can experience their best health and promote optimal brain function by eating mainly plant foods (75-80 percent) and a few choice animal foods (20-25 percent).

Organic eggs and cans of wild salmon are two of the most convenient and healthiest sources of animal protein and fat to have on hand.

Healthy Oils

- Virgin, organic coconut oil
- Cold-pressed, extra virgin olive oil in a dark bottle

Nutritional Supplements

- Cod liver oil or fish oil– this is the only nutritional supplement that I believe is an absolute must for optimal brain function and overall health. Nowhere else will you get an equally high quality, concentrated source of EPA and DHA, two long chain omega-3 fatty acids that are absolutely essential to the health of your brain and the rest of your nervous system. In addition to being necessary for optimal cognitive function, EPA and DHA are essential for promoting healthy mood regulation, which can only help you stick with your plan to be an effective student.

- A high quality probiotic – is not absolutely essential to optimal brain function like cod liver oil or fish oil are, but is very important for optimal digestion and a strong immune system, both of which indirectly support a healthy brain.

See: http://drbenkim.com/articles-probiotics.html to learn more about the health benefits of probiotics.

Foods that All Effective Students Need to Avoid

If you have a tiny portion of any of the foods listed below once in a great while, not to worry. The key is to stay away from the following foods as much as possible. These foods will put unnecessary stress on one or more of your major systems (digestive, nervous, cardiovascular, respiratory, immune, lymphatic, endocrine, and genito-urinary).

1. All deep fried foods. This includes French fries, fried chicken, tempura, donuts, and frozen foods that were originally made by deep-frying them.
2. Sugar and foods that contain sugar. You should also avoid all natural sugar substitutes like brown rice syrup, evaporated cane juice, and date sugar.
3. Margarine, shortening, and anything that has hydrogenated or partially hydrogenated oils.
4. Highly processed luncheon meats and sausage containing MSG and other additives.
5. Commercially processed foods such as cookies, cakes, crackers, donuts, TV dinners, soft drinks, packaged sauce mixes, etc.

6. Artificial food additives, especially MSG, and aspartame, which are neurotoxins. Most soups, sauces, broth mixes and commercial condiments contain MSG, even if not so labeled.
7. All vegetable oils made from soy, corn, safflower, sunflower, canola and cottonseed.
8. Pasteurized milk and all products made of pasteurized milk like cheese, butter, ice cream, whipped cream, cream cheese, coffee creamer, chocolate, and any baked goods or snacks that contain pasteurized milk. The only exceptions are organic yogurt and organic butter, which most non-Asian people can tolerate in small amounts without significant health problems.
9. All factory farmed (non-organic, non-free-range) animal products including beef, chicken, pork, eggs, and fish.
10. All non-fish seafood. This includes crab, lobster, shrimp, mussels, clams, oysters, and anything else that lives in water that is not fish.
11. Products that contain **isolated** protein, the most common forms being soy and whey.

12. Caffeine-containing beverages such as coffee, non-herbal tea, and soft drinks.

Strategy Number Eight:

Use Optimal Nutrition to Boost Your Brain Power

A One-Week Food Plan for Highly Effective Students

Before we get to the food plan, here are a few miscellaneous kitchen and food preparation tips:

- Use stainless steel cookware or corning ware. Avoid pots and pans that are made with aluminum or a stick-free coating like Teflon.
- Don't store your food in tin foil or pie or cake plates that are made out of aluminum.
- If you can tolerate dairy, always use unsalted butter. It is almost always more fresh than salted butter. If you must use some salt with your butter, use a mineral-dense sea salt.
- Use the smallest amount of dishwashing detergent possible, and rinse well with hot water. Many people eat dishwashing soap residues off their plates without knowing it.
- Don't use microwave ovens – there is more than enough experiential evidence out there to have me convinced that they can cause harmful changes to nutrients in food.
- Wash all of your fruits and vegetables thoroughly with water. If you want to be extra cautious, you can add some lemon juice and salt to a sink or basin full of water and use this

mixture to wash fruits and vegetables. Don't be afraid to get your hands right in there and rub your fruits and vegetables with water. Fruits like apples that have a waxy coating should be peeled.

- Consider buying a large container of baby field greens or baby spinach each week and keeping it in your refrigerator. Baby field greens and baby spinach are perfect for whole grain sandwiches and salads. Having them on hand will make it easy for you to make green vegetables the staple of your diet. Layer a few paper towels in between the greens and along the sides, bottom, and top of the container that they sit in; this will allow moisture that arises from the greens to be wicked away, which will keep the greens fresh for as long as possible.
- Soft boil six to twelve eggs over the weekend and keep them in your refrigerator, ready to eat at home or take with you to eat for lunch.
- If you are accustomed to using mayonnaise to make sandwiches for lunch, try switching to mustard, which provides tang and saltiness, but doesn't come with the harmful oil that

typically accompanies even the most expensive commercial brands of mayonnaise.

With the following one-week food plan, please don't ignore your own instincts. If a particular food or meal just doesn't appeal to you in the moment, try a different choice from another day. Feel free to be creative and mix and match some of the combinations. For example, if you feel like a different fruit or vegetable than the one that is suggested, by all means listen to your cravings. If you aren't so hungry on some days and feel like eating one or two meals instead of three, follow your instincts.

Please note that recipes for foods with an asterisk can be found in the resources section at the back of this book. Please don't forget to soak your whole grains, nuts, and dried fruit before preparing and eating.

One Week Food Plan

DAY 1

Breakfast
Organic eggs with tomato and avocado

Lunch
Large salad with dressing*, raw almonds, and avocado

Dinner
Can of wild salmon, steamed cabbage and broccoli, with dressing*

Snack
Apples

***

DAY 2

Breakfast
Any fresh fruit in season, bowl of oatmeal (soaked before preparing)

Lunch
Large vegetable sandwich made with whole grain bread, avocado, red onions, mustard, and a large handful of baby field greens or baby spinach

Dinner
Brown rice, black beans, guacamole*

Snack
Raw nuts (soaked)

***

DAY 3

Breakfast
Toasted whole grain pita with organic butter, two soft boiled eggs, tomato

Lunch
Gritty pita with cucumbers, hummus, avocado, and red onion

Dinner
Vegetable salad with dressing*, chickpea and leek soup, brown rice with avocado

Snack
Your choice of berries with organic yogurt if you can tolerate dairy. If you cannot tolerate dairy, just the berries.

***

DAY 4

Breakfast
Miso soup* with shredded bok choy or spinach, brown rice

Lunch
Vegetable salad with dressing*, baked corn chips, salsa, and guacamole*

Dinner
Salad, steamed zucchini and broccoli, organic turkey sausage with avocado

Snack
Green and black olives

***

DAY 5

Breakfast
Avocado, tomato, celery sticks, cucumber

Lunch
Vegetable salad with dressing*, olives and one soft boiled egg*

Dinner
Steamed zucchini, carrots, and green beans with black bean dip* and avocado

Snack
Classic berry smoothie*

***

Day 6

Breakfast
Watermelon with avocado, followed by raw cashews

Lunch
Gritty pita with tomato, avocado, cucumber, red onion, and a large handful of baby field greens or baby spinach

Dinner
Wild salmon (fresh or canned), steamed cabbage and broccoli, small salad with dressing*

Snack
Mango

***

Day 7

Breakfast
Apples, blueberries, romaine lettuce, celery, avocado

Lunch
Large salad with dressing*
1 can of wild salmon

Dinner
Steamed asparagus, broccoli, and green beans with dressing*
Brown rice with avocado

Snack
Walnuts with a few raisins

***

Be sure to check out the recipes section at the back of this book for more delicious and healthy meal and snack ideas. And remember to never underestimate the power your food choices have to influence your ability to be a clear-minded and effective learner.

If you would like more comprehensive guidance on how to be as healthy as possible, I recommend that you read ***Experience Your Best Health: A complete guide to taking care of your health from the inside out***. You can learn more about this book at:

http://drbenkim.com/experience-your-best-health.html

A Priceless Lesson That I Learned from a Professional Tennis Player

Towards the end of my days as a chiropractic student in the suburbs of Chicago, I was thrilled to find out that there would be a professional women's tennis tournament in Chicago. The top players at the time – Martina Hingis, Jana Novotna, and Lindsay Davenport – were all scheduled to be there. Being a huge tennis fan and avid player ever since I first started playing in elementary school, I was psyched at the opportunity to watch these incredible athletes up close.

A friend of mine told me that I would have a lot more fun watching the players practice than I would watching them play actual matches. I wasn't sure how this could be, but since it was a once in a lifetime opportunity, I followed my friend's advice and made my way down to the venue three hours before matches were scheduled to start.

To put it simply, the experience of watching these gifted athletes practice was inspiring and amazing. When Martina Hingis first came out onto the court, she kept her warm-up jacket on and took tiny little baby steps up and down the court, about as fast as a baby can crawl. She then did the same thing with side to side shuffle steps for several minutes. I was amazed that this 16 year old, world class athlete took the time to warm up with such precision.

After another 15 minutes of warming up in an equally methodical and painfully-slow-to-watch fashion, she moved to the middle of the court, right by the net, with her hitting partner, where the two of them begin hitting balls back and forth with such softness and grace that it looked like they were under water. No grunting or magnificent displays of power like I was used to watching on TV. Slowly, over several minutes, they both gradually inched backwards to their respective ends of the court and began hitting with the longer and more powerful strokes that I was used to seeing on TV.

What I found particularly impressive was how they would use the exact same stroke to hit to the exact same location over and over again before moving to a different stroke and location.

Fifty waist-high forehands cross court.

Fifty shoulder-high forehands cross court.

Fifty waist-high forehands down the line.

Fifty shoulder-high forehands down the line.

The same series of shots except with the backhand.

You get the picture, right? They were so finely trained that it looked like they were on automatic pilot, with their rippling muscles and reactive tendons capable of putting the ball within inches of wherever they wanted, every single time!

The ultimate highlight came at the end of the practice session. Martina Hingis was practicing overhead smashes at the net. She must have hit about twenty of them when her mother and coach,

Melanie Molitor yelled out, "Okay!" meaning that Martina could wrap it up. But just before her mother had yelled out, Martina's hitting partner had hit another lob for Martina to smash down with another overhead stroke. Even though Martina's right hand (her strong hand) was up and cocked back, ready to smash the ball, when she heard her mom's signal to end the practice session, with the ball in mid-flight and coming towards her, she casually switched her racket from her right hand to her weaker left hand, and smashed the ball cross court with as much power and grace as she had showed all along with her strong side! I remember being so stunned that my jaw literally dropped open. Being really into a bunch of sports since I was young, I knew full well how hard it was to perform with the same strength and grace on one's weak side, leg or arm. That one spontaneous, playful smash with her left hand was the exclamation mark on my realization of how extraordinary her talent and training was.

Why have I shared this story in a book about how to be an effective learner and the best student you can be? Because in case you aren't already aware of this, I want you to know what kind of dedication it takes to be extraordinary in any area of your life. Not all of us have the genetics and life circumstances to allow us to develop into professional athletes or achieve the highest grades in our classes. But all of us *do* have a chance to dedicate ourselves to doing the very best we can in school and life.

Legendary basketball coach, John Wooden, defines success as follows:

Success is peace of mind that can only be attained by knowing that you did the best you could with your God-given talents.

As John Wooden points out in his autobiography, you can fool your parents, teachers, and friends, but you can't fool yourself. At the end of each day, you know deep in your heart if you have done your best. And if you haven't, you will fall short of having peace of mind. And without peace of mind, no matter how much money you make, what kind of car you drive, and how beautiful your house is, you are almost guaranteed to feel like a failure deep in your heart.

Now, I'm not suggesting that you should live your life surrounded by textbooks. I believe that doing your best in school is healthiest in the context of striving to live a well balanced life that feels meaningful to you. How can you know if you are living a meaningful life? Imagine that we all had only five years left to live. What would you do with your last five years?

Here are a few suggestions:

Have fun with your family and friends. Show your loved ones how much you care about them though your daily behavior. Play with your dog. Enjoy an afternoon nap. Make yourself and others a delicious snack. Read books that inspire and motivate you, or just make you plain happy. Look for ways that you can encourage others. Work on being a person who keeps her promises and has a reputation of being trustworthy. Work at not gossiping about others, ever. Be creative and work on projects that you are excited about. And when you make time to study, study the right way, a way that feels right for you and hopefully incorporates some or all of the suggestions in this book.

When you strive to live a meaningful life, you will consistently feel peace of mind, and this will only make it easier for you to be the best student you can be.

Healthy and Delicious Recipes

Delicious and Nutritious Dressings and Dips

Super Simple Dressing Recipe

2 tablespoons of cold pressed, extra virgin olive oil
2 teaspoons of vinegar or freshly squeezed lemon juice
1-3 teaspoons of raw, unheated honey, to taste
1 teaspoon of mustard
Sea salt, to taste

Use a fork to whisk all ingredients together in a small bowl. Pour over a vegetable salad in a large bowl. Toss to evenly coat vegetables with dressing and enjoy.

Broccoli-Tahini Dressing Recipe

2 large stalks of broccoli
2 tablespoons of raw tahini
Spring water
Sea salt, to taste

Steam broccoli until bright green and slightly tender. Combine steamed broccoli and raw tahini in a blender with spring water and blend until desired consistency is reached. Add sea salt, to taste.

Enjoy this rich and delicious dressing over other steamed vegetables or a whole grain dish.

This recipe was adapted from a similar recipe found in the May/June 1999 issue of Health Science.

Miso-Walnut Dressing Recipe

This Asian-style dressing goes beautifully with pasta, brown rice, quinoa, any steamed vegetables, and even a fresh, crunchy salad. You can find high quality miso at any Asian food market and most health food stores. All Korean markets carry den-jang, a Korean version of miso that works just as well with this recipe.

2 tablespoons of miso
1/3 cup of fresh, raw walnuts
1/4 cup of sesame oil
1 tablespoon of unpasteurized or raw honey
2 1/2 tablespoons of brown rice vinegar

Blend all ingredients together in a food processor until smooth. If you like a thinner consistency, add a little water. Serve immediately or after chilling for an hour in the refrigerator.

Tahini Dressing Recipe
2 heaping tablespoons of raw, organic tahini
1/2 clove of garlic
Juice of 1/4 of a lemon
Sea salt, to taste
Water

Blend all ingredients, adding water slowly until desired consistency is reached. This creamy dressing is perfect for salads, steamed vegetables, and sandwiches.

House Dressing Recipe
1/2 cup of cold-pressed, extra virgin olive oil
2 and 1/2 tablespoons of freshly squeezed lemon juice
1 teaspoon of Dijon mustard
Sea salt, to taste
Black pepper, to taste

Mix mustard and lemon juice in a bowl. Add olive oil in a slow, steady stream while mixing. Add sea salt and black pepper, to taste. Enjoy this dressing over a fresh salad, steamed vegetables, or whole grains.

Mango Avocado Dressing Recipe
1 ripe avocado
1 ripe mango
1/2 lemon, freshly squeezed
Sea salt (optional)

Blend all ingredients and serve immediately over salad, steamed vegetables, or whole grain dish. Enjoy this bright and refreshing salad dressing recipe.

Creamy Sunflower Dressing Recipe
1 cup of raw sunflower seeds
1/2 clove of garlic
Juice of 1/4 of a lemon
1 teaspoon of raw honey (optional)
Sea salt, to taste
Water

Blend all ingredients, adding water slowly until desired consistency is reached. This creamy dressing will bring any vegetable salad or plate of steamed vegetables alive. Enjoy.

Unforgettable Guacamole Recipe
1 ripe avocado
1/5 of a whole red onion, chopped
Juice of 1/2 of a lemon or lime
1/4 cup of fresh cilantro, chopped
Sea salt, to taste

Scoop flesh of ripe avocado into a large bowl. Add all other ingredients and mash with a fork. If you want good texture, don't mash too much - just enough to evenly distribute the ingredients and break down the avocado into chunky portions.

This has got to be one of our all-time favourite snacks. Try it with baked corn chips and be prepared to make some more.

Creamy Hummus Recipe
1 can of chickpeas, or 2 cups of dry chickpeas
1 tablespoon of raw, organic tahini
1 clove of garlic
Juice of 1 small lemon
1/4 chopped red onion (optional)
Sea salt, to taste
Extra virgin olive oil

Rinse and bring canned chickpeas to a boil for one minute to help remove preservatives. If you use dry chickpeas, soak them in water overnight and cook for about an hour or until tender over medium heat.

After warming up chickpeas in a pot of boiling water and draining them, combine chickpeas and all other ingredients except olive oil in a food processor. As the ingredients blend together, add olive oil until desired consistency is reached.

Try this delicious, creamy hummus with toasted whole grain bread, sliced tomatoes, and lettuce. It is best served warm, but keeps well in an airtight container for several days in the refrigerator.

Note: You can make a **Black Bean Dip** with this hummus recipe by substituting the chickpeas with black beans.

Soups

Traditional Korean Seaweed Soup Recipe
1 package of dried seaweed (1 ounce is fine for four servings), available in all Korean food markets
6 cups of vegetable broth or organic chicken broth
2 teaspoons of sesame oil
Naturally brewed soy sauce or sea salt, to taste
1 teaspoon of minced garlic (optional)

Soak seaweed in water for two hours or until soft. Drain and rinse really well, as dried seaweed can come with a lot of dirt, just like spinach does.

Put all ingredients, including seaweed, into a large pot and bring to a boil, then simmer for five minutes to allow all the flavors to come together.

Koreans traditionally enjoy this seaweed soup with a bowl of white or brown rice, sometimes together in the same bowl.

Vegetable Broth Recipe
1 whole onion, halved
3 ribs of celery, chopped
3 carrots, chopped
1 zucchini, chopped
3 potatoes, chopped
Any leftover greens like Swiss chard, beet tops, or turnip tops, chopped
Sea salt, to taste

Combine all vegetables in a large pot. Fill with spring or filtered water until vegetables are fully covered. Bring to a boil. Lower heat and leave it to simmer with the lid on for one hour.
Strain well. Add sea salt, to taste.

Simple Pea Soup Recipe
8 cups frozen peas
5 cups vegetable or chicken broth
1 garlic clove, roughly chopped
2 tablespoons of organic butter
Sea salt and black pepper, to taste

Over medium to high heat, cook garlic in butter for 2-3 minutes. Add peas and cook for an additional 1-2 minutes.

Add vegetable or chicken broth, bring to a boil, then reduce heat to allow ingredients to simmer for 5 minutes with the lid on.

Blend all ingredients in a food processor until smooth and return to pot. Add sea salt and black pepper, to taste.

If available, garnish with a sprig of fresh mint. Enjoy this healthy and simple pea soup recipe.

Black Bean Soup Recipe
For this recipe, you will need to soak 3 cups of dry black beans in water overnight. After soaking, cook beans in water over medium heat for 1-2 hours or until tender.

3 cups cooked black beans
2 cups vegetable broth or water
1 carrot, finely chopped
1 rib of celery, finely chopped
1 yellow onion, finely chopped
2 cloves of garlic, finely minced or pressed
2 tablespoons of fresh lemon juice
Handful of fresh parsley, chopped
Sea salt and black pepper, to taste

Combine all ingredients except lemon juice, parsley, sea salt, and black pepper in a large pot and cook until vegetables are tender. Puree mixture in a blender or a food processor until creamy. Return to pot. Add lemon juice, parsley, sea salt, and pepper. You can serve this yummy soup immediately or freeze it for later.

Hearty Chickpea and Leek Soup Recipe
1 can of chickpeas or two cups of dry chickpeas
2 leeks (most grocery stores sell them in groups of 3)
1 small potato

Vegetable broth
Sea salt and pepper, to taste (optional)

If you use a can of chickpeas, rinse them well and bring them to a boil for a minute to help get rid of any preservatives. If you use dry chickpeas, soak them in water overnight and cook them over medium heat for about an hour or until tender.

Cut leeks in half lengthwise and soak in water to remove dirt. Chop leeks and potato into bite-size pieces and boil them in just enough water to cover them for about 10 minutes or until tender.

Add chickpeas and allow all ingredients to sit on low heat for a minute or two.

Blend ingredients in a food processor or blender. Return blended mixture to pot, and add vegetable broth until desired consistency is reached. Season with sea salt if desired.

Traditional Korean Miso Soup Recipe
This delicious and nourishing miso soup is a great way to enjoy the benefits of fermented soy. It is a staple in the traditional Korean diet.

You can find Korean miso - called ***den jang*** - at your local Korean supermarket. If you don't have a Korean market in your area, you can use a Japanese version of miso, found at any Asian food market or your local health food store.
2 tablespoons of den jang or miso
1 yellow onion, peeled and chopped
1 zucchini, chopped into bite-size pieces
Small handful of dried anchovies, found at your local Asian market (optional)
4 cups of spring or filtered water

Boil onions and anchovies in 4 cups of water for five minutes or until onions become tender. Reduce heat to between low and medium and add zucchini and den jang or miso. Use a spoon to help dissolve the den jang or miso into the water by spreading it along the inside of your pot. As soon as den jang or miso is dissolved, take off heat and serve.

This traditional Korean miso soup is usually served with a side bowl of brown rice and one or two side dishes of vegetables. Depending on how sensitive your sense of taste is, you may need to add more or less den jang or miso.

Cabbage Chickpea Soup Recipe
2 cups chopped cabbage
1 can chickpeas, rinsed and drained
1 large Yukon gold potato
1 onion, chopped
2 garlic cloves, pressed
1/4 cup cilantro, finely chopped
4 cups of filtered or spring water or Vegetable Broth
Sea salt and black pepper, to taste

Use 4 cups of water or vegetable broth to boil all ingredients except cilantro, salt, and pepper. Boil until vegetables are tender.
Transfer 3 cups of soup into a blender and blend until creamy.
Add blended mixture back to pot, adding cilantro, salt and pepper to taste.
Stir for a minute and serve.

This soup is great by itself or with a bowl of rice and a fresh vegetable salad.

Broccoli Potato Soup Recipe
2 onions, chopped
5 cups vegetable broth or water

6 potatoes, diced
2 large broccoli heads, chopped into florets. Broccoli stems skinned and sliced
1 garlic clove, minced or pressed
2 and 1/2 tablespoons of fresh lemon juice
Sea salt and black pepper, to taste

Combine onions, vegetable broth or water, potatoes, and broccoli in a large pot and cook until vegetables are tender. Puree mixture in a blender or a food processor until creamy. Return to pot. Add lemon juice, garlic, sea salt, and pepper. Enjoy this nutritious and filling soup.

Savoury Squash Soup Recipe
2 large acorn or 1 butternut squash
1 large Spanish or any yellow onion, roughly chopped
1 clove of garlic, finely chopped
3 cups of vegetable broth
Sea salt, to taste (optional)

Cut squash into halves and place skin side down in a casserole dish. Cover with foil and bake at 375 degrees Fahrenheit, or until tender. After it cools enough for you to handle, scoop out the flesh.

In a fair sized pot, boil onions and garlic in vegetable broth until tender. Add the cooked squash and sea salt. Blend all ingredients with a hand held blender or in a conventional blender if you like a smooth, creamy soup.

Healthy Drinks

Cleansing and Nourishing Vegetable Juices

2 carrots
2 ribs of celery
8 leaves of romaine lettuce

2 carrots
Handful of parsley
6 leaves of romaine lettuce
Squeeze of lemon

2 tomatoes
3 ribs of celery
1 carrot
Squeeze of lemon

6 leaves of romaine lettuce
1 tomato
1 rib of celery
1 carrot

Big bunch of kale
2 carrots
2 ribs of celery
Big bunch of Swiss chard
2 carrots
2 ribs of celery

6 leaves of romaine lettuce
2 cups of green cabbage
2 carrots

All-Natural Almond Milk Recipe
1 ½ cups of raw almonds, soaked in water overnight
4 cups of filtered or spring water
3-5 dates (optional)

Blend 1 ½ cups of raw almonds that have been soaked overnight in 4 cups of water. Blend with dates if you like your milk with a hint of sweetness. Strain once to remove almond granules. The result is delicious, creamy milk that is free of harmful vegetable oil, concentrated sweeteners, and the problems associated with cow's milk and soy. It can be stored safely for 3-4 days in the refrigerator.

Banana Peanut Butter Smoothie Recipe
2 small bananas
1 tablespoon of organic, all-natural peanut butter
1 cup of almond milk or spring water

Blend all ingredients and enjoy.

Power Shake Recipe
One of the most nutritious foods that many people can eat are raw, organic eggs. If you use eggs that are produced by birds that are free to roam around on a farm, you do not have to worry about dangerous pathogens. Keep in mind that raw, organic eggs have been eaten for thousands of years by many different cultures throughout Europe and Asia. Russians and Koreans are particularly fond of them.

You won't even taste the eggs in this delicious and nutritious shake.

2 organic eggs
1 banana
2 tablespoons of frozen blueberries
1/3 cup of water or almond milk

Blend all ingredients for 20 seconds and enjoy this power shake.

Classic Berry Smoothie
1 frozen banana, halved or chunked
2-3 tablespoons of frozen or thawed wild blueberries
1 handful of strawberries
1 cup of almond milk or 1 cup of water with 10 raw almonds

Blend all ingredients until desired consistency is reached. This smoothie is best if you drink it while you're barefoot and looking at the sky or some trees.

Salads

Mediterranean Salad Recipe

4 cups of flat or curled parsley, chopped
1 large or 2 medium cucumbers, peeled and chopped into bite-size pieces
1 rib of celery, finely chopped
1 tomato, finely chopped
1/2 cup of your favourite olives
2 tablespoons of freshly squeezed lemon juice
3 tablespoons of cold-pressed extra virgin olive oil
Sea salt and black pepper, to taste

Put parsley, cucumbers, celery, olives, and tomatoes into a bowl. Mix all other ingredients and pour over salad. Toss well. If you can tolerate organic goat's cheese, sprinkle some on top. Enjoy this healthy meal from the Mediterranean.

Avocado Orange Salad Recipe

2 ripe avocados, scooped out and cut into bite-size pieces
2 oranges, peeled and sectioned
2-4 leaves of dark green lettuce like romaine or red leaf
1 tablespoon of chopped green onions (optional)
House Dressing, to taste

Put avocado and oranges on a plate lined with lettuce, sprinkle with chopped green onions, and add dressing. Enjoy this simple and delicious salad.

Carrot and Jicama Salad Recipe

This crunchy and tasty salad is best made with a good vegetable shredder called a mandolin. If you don't have a mandolin but want to buy one, try your local Asian food supermarket. Almost all Korean supermarkets carry an excellent one for around twenty-five dollars.

Jicama is a white-fleshed root vegetable that is a good source of vitamin C. It adds a great crunchy component to salads.

3 small carrots, peeled and shredded
1 small to medium jicama, peeled and shredded
1 yellow or red bell pepper, seeded and sliced into thin strips
1/4 red onion, sliced into thin strips
1 cup of chopped cilantro
House Dressing, to taste

Combine all ingredients in a large salad bowl, add house dressing, and toss. Enjoy this crunchy, healthy, and yummy salad.

Egg Salad with Artichokes Recipe
5 soft-boiled organic eggs, peeled and chopped into bite-size pieces
1 can of artichoke hearts, drained and chopped into bite-size pieces
1 small tomato, chopped
1/2 avocado, chopped
1 small green onion, chopped
House Dressing, to taste

Combine all ingredients in a large bowl and stir gently. Serve immediately and enjoy this delicious and healthy egg salad.

Main and Side Dishes

Avocado-Potato Salad Recipe
1 large ripe avocado, mashed
6 medium Yukon gold or red potatoes
1/2 cup chopped red onion
2 ribs of celery, chopped
1/2 cup sweet red bell pepper
Sea salt, to taste

Steam and cook the potatoes until tender but not too soft. Mix thoroughly with all other ingredients. Keep refrigerated until ready to serve. Enjoy this simple and delicious avocado-potato salad.

This recipe was adapted from a similar recipe found in the May/June 1999 issue of Health Science.

Cold Korean Noodles with Sesame Dressing Recipe

1/4 cup vegetable broth
3 tablespoons unpasteurized honey
2 tablespoons organic tahini
1 tablespoon rice wine vinegar
1 tablespoon sesame oil
1 tablespoon naturally brewed soy sauce or tamari
1 teaspoon minced garlic
8 oz. buckwheat noodles (rice noodles or regular pasta noodles will do if you can't find buckwheat noodles)
1 cup asparagus cut into bite-size pieces
1 cup chopped red bell peppers
1 cup chopped broccoli
1/2 cup chopped green onions

Use a food processor to blend stock, honey, tahini, vinegar, sesame oil, soy sauce, and garlic. Set aside.

Boil buckwheat noodles until ready to eat. Drain and rinse with cold water. Put into a big bowl.
Steam or boil asparagus and broccoli for about 1 minute. Rinse with cold water, drain, and add to noodles. Add red bell peppers and green onions.

Pour dressing over noodles and vegetables and toss well. Serve and enjoy immediately.

Note: If you make this dish ahead of time, don't mix the dressing with the vegetables and noodles until right before you serve.

Margaret's Mushroom & Sweet Brown Rice Risotto Recipe

5 cups button mushrooms, sliced thin
1 medium onion, chopped
1 cup sweet brown rice, uncooked
5 and a half cups chicken or vegetable broth
Sea salt to taste
2 tablespoons olive oil

1. Cook the rice in a covered pot in 2 and a half cups of the broth. Wait until it's fully cooked before doing anything else. The rice is done when it's soft. The cooked grains should stick together slightly, as it is sweet brown rice.

2. In a medium or large pot, sauté the onion in the olive oil. When onion is soft, add the mushrooms and a pinch of sea salt.

3. When the mushrooms are soft, add the cooked rice and sea salt to taste. Add the rest of the broth (3 cups) and mix until everything is well-incorporated.

This recipe serves 2 - 3 people. Enjoy!

Thai Vegetable Scramble Recipe

1 tablespoon Virgin Coconut Oil
1/3 small zucchini, finely chopped
1/4 small onion, finely chopped
1/3 small red bell pepper, chopped
1-2 organic eggs
Sea salt and black pepper, to taste

In a small pan, melt the coconut oil. Add the zucchini, onions, and red bell pepper and sauté until tender.

Whisk eggs gently in a small bowl. Add salt and pepper to taste.
Pour eggs into the pan when the vegetables are tender and scramble lightly.
Serve immediately and enjoy this simple and delicious Thai recipe.

Pea and Mint Omelette Recipe
1/2 cup frozen peas
3 organic eggs
1 tablespoon chopped fresh mint
1 tablespoon of organic butter, coconut oil, or olive oil
Sea salt and black pepper, to taste

Boil peas in water for a couple of minutes or until tender. Be sure not to cook so long that you lose their bright green color. Drain well and keep to side.

Beat eggs with a fork in a medium to large bowl. Add peas, mint, sea salt, and pepper.

Melt butter in a large pan over medium heat. Add egg mixture, doing your best to evenly distribute mixture in pan. Use your spatula to move uncooked portions of egg towards the edges of your pan from time to time to ensure even cooking. If you are unable to cook eggs evenly before you get too much browning on the underside of your omelet, finish off cooking in your oven with the broiler setting for a minute or two.

Coconut Curry Recipe
1 tablespoon virgin coconut oil
1 can of coconut milk* (1 1/2 or 2 cans if you like curry with more sauce)
1 teaspoon chopped garlic
2 pinches of sea salt, or to taste
4 large potatoes, peeled and chopped
1/2 head large cauliflower, chopped
2 cups zucchini, chopped

2 tablespoons curry powder
1/2 teaspoon ground cumin
1/2 teaspoon ground nutmeg
1/2 teaspoon ground ginger

In a bowl, stir together the curry powder, cumin, nutmeg, and ginger.

Steam potatoes for 20 minutes, adding cauliflower for the last 5 minutes. Heat coconut oil in a large saucepan. Add garlic and zucchini. Cook until zucchini softens a bit. Add the steamed potatoes and cauliflower to the saucepan. Add coconut milk. Stir in the spices and salt. Continue stirring until spices are incorporated. Serve by itself or over brown rice or quinoa.

Serves five.

*Most grocery stores now carry canned coconut milk that contains 0.003% or zero preservatives. If you cannot find a good source at your local supermarket, try visiting a Chinese grocery store.

Quinoa and Vegetable Salad Recipe
If you aren't familiar with quinoa (pronounced keen-wa), you're in for a treat. Quinoa is a light and fluffy whole grain that goes with just about anything. It's power packed with protein, iron, potassium, and several B vitamins. It's also a good source of magnesium, zinc, copper, and manganese, and has some folic acid.

1 cup of quinoa
1/2 cucumber, peeled and chopped into bite-size pieces
1 tomato, chopped into bite size pieces
1 avocado, seeded, scooped out, and cut into small pieces

Juice of 1/2 to 1 lemon
Sea salt, to taste

Combine quinoa in a pot with 2 cups of spring or filtered water. Bring to a boil, then keep on low heat with lid on. Check occasionally. When you don't see any water in the pot, it's done. Allow quinoa to cool in a large salad bowl for around 15 minutes.

Add all chopped vegetables to quinoa. Add lemon juice. Add salt, if desired. Toss well, and enjoy this hearty and healthy grain salad.

Sweet and Sour Cabbage and Beans Recipe
This is one of our favourite dishes. Try serving it piping hot over brown rice or quinoa.

1 can of beans, organic if possible
1 1/2 C tomato sauce
6 C shredded cabbage
1 tablespoon lemon juice
1 teaspoon apple cider vinegar
3 tablespoons honey
1 teaspoon Dijon mustard
1/4 C raisins
1 medium onion chopped
1 large clove of garlic chopped
Place all ingredients except beans in a large saucepan, bring to the boil and then cover and simmer for 10 min. Add the beans and cook until warmed.

Soft Boiled Eggs Recipe
I know it seems almost silly to have a recipe for boiled eggs, but I have found that many people boil their eggs for too long, decreasing the quality of protein and fat that properly cooked and raw eggs provide.

Here's how to boil an egg to preserve as much of its health benefits as possible:

Place your eggs in a pot and add enough cold water to completely cover eggs. Allow this pot to sit on medium to medium-high heat until the water is just ready to boil. At this point, put a lid on the pot and take it off the heat completely, allowing it to rest on a part of your stove that is at room temperature. After 15 minutes, rinse well with lukewarm or room temperature water and peel. Voila - tasty and nutritious soft boiled eggs!

Traditional Korean Miso Wrap Recipe

The star of this recipe is a paste made out of den jang (Korean version of miso), a touch of hot chili paste, and sesame oil. Koreans call this paste ***sahm jang***. If you cannot find den jang, feel free to use miso as a substitute.

1 tablespoon of den jang or miso
1 1/2 teaspoons of sesame oil
1/4 teaspoon of hot chili paste

Mix ingredients together in a small bowl until uniform. Sahm jang is served in its own bowl at the center of the table, with a large plate of fresh romaine lettuce or red leaf lettuce leaves, and a bowl of brown rice for each person.

Place a small spoonful of brown rice in the center of a piece of lettuce, add a small dollop of sahm jang to the rice, wrap closed with the outer portions of the lettuce, and enjoy! Two people will typically need a whole head of romaine lettuce leaves for one meal.

Pesto Salmon Recipe

1 1/4 cups loosely packed fresh basil
1 clove garlic

3 tablespoons vegetable or chicken broth
1 tablespoon blanched slivered almonds
1 tablespoon lemon juice
2 teaspoons freshly grated Parmesan cheese (optional)
2 teaspoons extra-virgin olive oil
1/4 teaspoon sea salt
1/4 teaspoon freshly ground black pepper
1 pound skinned pacific wild salmon fillet, cut into 4 pieces
lemon wedges (optional)
basil sprigs (optional)

Place the basil, garlic, broth, almonds, lemon juice, cheese, oil, sea salt, and pepper in a blender and process until pureed.

Place salmon on a plate. Spoon 3 tablespoons of the pesto over salmon and turn to coat both sides. Cover with plastic wrap and let stand for 15 minutes. Keep remaining pesto on the side.

Meanwhile, preheat the broiler and lightly oil a pan or baking sheet.

Place salmon in prepared pan. Broil salmon 4" to 5" from the heat for 6 to 8 minutes, or just until opaque.

Place salmon pieces on 4 plates and top each piece with some of the reserved pesto. Garnish with lemon wedges and basil sprigs, if available.

Deluxe Veggie Sandwich Recipe
1/2 ripe avocado. sliced
Few slices of red onion
1 leaf of romaine lettuce
2 slices of tomato
Small bunch of sprouts, any kind (optional)

2 slices of whole grain bread, toasted
Dijon mustard, to taste

Pile all vegetables and Dijon mustard in between two slices of toasted whole grain bread. Chew to liquid and enjoy this filling and healthy deluxe veggie sandwich recipe.

Green Beans, Korean Style Recipe
1 pound (2-3 large handfuls) fresh green beans, washed, trimmed, and cut in half
1 medium onion, cut in half and then sliced into thin strips
1/3 cup water or Vegetable Broth
1 tablespoon naturally brewed soy sauce
1 tablespoon rice vinegar

Steam green beans until tender - around 8-12 minutes.
While green beans are steaming, cook onion over medium heat with water or vegetable broth in a large pan. Cook for 5 minutes or until tender. Turn the heat to between low and medium and add rice vinegar and soy sauce. Add green beans and toss slightly to mix green beans in with onions. Cook green beans and onions together for 2-3 minutes to allow soy sauce and vinegar to evenly coat all vegetables. Try serving these yummy Korean style green beans over a bowl of brown or white rice.

Vegetable and Goat's Cheese Pizza Recipe
Pizza Crust Ingredients:
1/2 cup warm water
2 1/4 cups whole wheat flour
1 teaspoon salt
1 tablespoon olive oil, plus more for spreading

Pizza Topping Ingredients:
1 tablespoon olive oil

Pinch of sea salt
4 cups tomato sauce
1 head broccoli, cut into small pieces
1 zucchini, diced
1 orange bell pepper, diced
1 onion, diced
2 cloves of garlic, finely chopped
Goat cheese, to taste

In a large bowl, mix together the flour and salt. Stir in 1 tablespoon olive oil, and the 1/2 cup of water until combined. Turn the dough out onto a work surface and knead until smooth (about 3 minutes). If the dough is too moist, you may need to add some flour to the work surface.

When you are ready to make the pizza, preheat the oven to 350 degrees Fahrenheit. Roll out the dough using a rolling pin. You may roll out the entire mound of dough for one pizza, or split the mound into two parts for two smaller pizzas. Place the rolled out dough on a lightly oiled baking sheet or pizza pan and bake for 10 minutes. Take the baked dough out of the oven and let rest while you prepare the toppings.

For the toppings, heat the olive oil in a large frying pan. Add the onions, garlic, broccoli, and bell pepper. Sauté for 3-5 minutes. Add the zucchini and pinch of salt. Sauté for another 2 minutes.

Spread the tomato sauce on the baked pizza dough so that it comes within a 1/2 inch of the edge.

Spread the toppings, plus the goat cheese if desired, on the pizza.

Put the pizza(s) back into the 350 degree Fahrenheit oven for 5-10 minutes. Serve hot and enjoy this healthy and delicious pizza.

Desserts and Snacks

Papaya with Lime Recipe

When choosing a papaya, look for one that has a nice yellow color and smells like papaya.

Cut ripe papaya in half, scoop out seeds, and cut into bite-size pieces. Squeeze fresh lime juice over papaya chunks. Enjoy this refreshing, sweet and sour treat.

Honeydew with Lemon Recipe

A ripe honeydew usually has a very mild yellow tinge to its skin and smells like fresh melon.

Cut ripe honeydew in half, scoop out seeds, and cut into chunks. Squeeze fresh lemon juice over honeydew and eat immediately.

Better than Candy Date Pecan Ball Recipe

2 cups of raw pecans
1 and 1/2 cups of dates
Spring or filtered water

Soak pecans and dates for 1-2 hours in water. Drain well and blend together in a food processor or strong blender until it turns into a coarse paste. Use your hands to form paste into bite-size balls. Enjoy these delicious treats right away, or save them in a container in the refrigerator for later. They keep well for up to three days in the refrigerator.

Save these date pecan balls for occasional treats, as dates are extremely concentrated in sugar and can contribute to health problems if eaten in large amounts.

Sunflower Raisin Cookie Recipe

3 cups soaked, raw sunflower seeds (soaked overnight)
10 pitted dates

1 cup chopped, dried, pre-soaked apricots
1 cup pre-soaked raisins (2 hours), drained on a dish towel
1 cup almond butter
1 tablespoon vanilla (optional)
1/2 teaspoon cinnamon (optional)

Blend all ingredients in food processor to a nutty consistency. Roll into small balls and flatten out to about 1/4 inch thickness. Cover and refrigerate for one hour before serving.

From the Fall 2001 edition of Health Science Magazine

Crispy Pecans Recipe
4 cups raw pecans
2 teaspoons sea salt
Spring or filtered water

Combine all ingredients in a large bowl and mix well. You should use enough water to fully cover pecans plus about two inches of extra water above the pecans. Leave mixture to sit overnight or for eight hours.

Drain mixture well with a colander and spread pecans out on a large cookie tray.

Keep tray in a warm oven (less than 150 degrees Fahrenheit) for 12 hours or until completely dry and crisp. Be sure to turn the pecans a few times during this time.

Store in an airtight container.

I know that this seems like a lot of work for a few crispy nuts, but once you try them, you'll probably be making more.

By the way, you can do the exact same thing with other nuts like almonds and organic peanuts.

For more delicious and healthy recipe ideas, please feel free to visit:

http://drbenkim.com/recipes.html

Did you borrow this book?

If you want to own a copy yourself or buy it as a gift for someone, you can place an order at http://drbenkim.com

For information on discounts for orders of 10 or more books, you can e-mail us at info@drbenkim.com.